C000006098

PLANT-BASED COOKBOOK

*Living In Harmony With Nature Thanks to
Amazing Plant Based Recipes*

GREEN KITCHEN

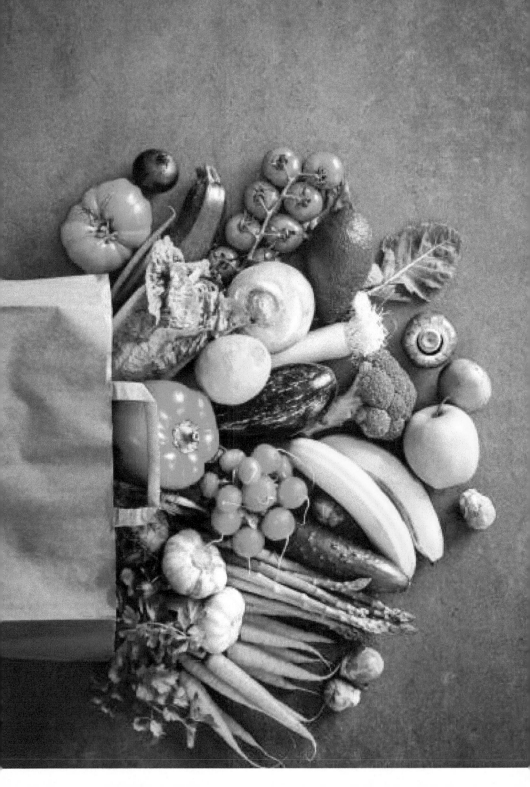

© Copyright 2021 by Green Kitchen- All rights reserved.

The following Book is reproduced below with the goal of providing information that is as accurate and reliable as possible. Regardless, purchasing this Book can be seen as consent to the fact that both the publisher and the author of this book are in no way experts on the topics discussed within and that any recommendations or suggestions that are made herein are for entertainment purposes only. Professionals should be consulted as needed prior to undertaking any of the action endorsed herein.

This declaration is deemed fair and valid by both the American Bar Association and the Committee of Publishers Association and is legally binding throughout the United States.
Furthermore, the transmission, duplication, or reproduction of any of the following work including specific information will be considered an illegal act irrespective of if it is done electronically or in print. This extends to creating a secondary or tertiary copy of the work or a recorded copy and is only allowed with the express written consent from the Publisher. All additional right reserved.

The information in the following pages is broadly considered a truthful and accurate account of facts and as such, any inattention, use, or misuse of the information in question by the reader will render any resulting actions solely under their purview. There are no scenarios in which the publisher or the original author of this work can be in any fashion deemed liable for any hardship or damages that may befall them after undertaking information described herein.

Additionally, the information in the following pages is intended only for informational purposes and should thus be thought of as universal. As befitting its nature, it is presented without assurance regarding its prolonged validity or interim quality. Trademarks that are mentioned are done without written consent and can in no way be considered an endorsement from the trademark holder.

Table of Contents

INTRODUCTION

Eating healthy cannot be overemphasized, in a world where fast food and junk food is always available. We all know that we could and should be eating healthier but there are so many diets being advertised that it's hard to know what's best for you.

We're always reading about how processed foods are bad for your body. You may have also been advised repeatedly to avoid foods high in preservatives; however, no one likes to eat bland food or spend their time reading labels. This book will teach you how to find nutritious, delicious foods that will keep you satisfied while improving your health.

BENEFITS OF A BALANCED DIET

Before we dive into talking about the recipes and foods you need for a balanced diet, let's discuss a little more on the need for eating balanced diet regularly.

- IMPROVED MEMORY: I know what you are thinking. "Are you being serious right now? If I just eat a few vegetables, I can be like Einstein?" Yes! You may not be as smart as Einstein, but healthy nutrients like Vitamins D, E, and C will help improve brain functionality.

- PREVENTS CANCER: According to medical experts, eating food that contains antioxidant can help protect cells from damage, thereby leading to a reduction in the risk of getting cancer. Cancer can also be treated at its early stage with healthy food.

- EMOTIONAL STABILITY: I know what you are thinking again. "Do you mean that if I'm going through a heartbreak and I eat some healthy food, I will be better?"

Yeah! It's not quite as straightforward as that, but healthy meals help improve your moods and balance your emotions. Scientists and researchers in 2016 found out that meals with a high glycemic load (high in carbohydrates) can trigger symptoms of depression and fatigue. Vegetables and fruits have a lower glycemic load and will help keep your blood sugar balanced.

- WEIGHT LOSS: Being overweight or obese can lead to other complicated illnesses like heart diseases, loss of bone density, and some types of cancer. Maintaining a healthful diet free from processed foods can help you stay at a healthy weight without resorting to fad diets.

- STRONG BONES AND TEETH: For healthy bones and teeth, a diet rich in calcium and magnesium is important. Maintaining bone integrity can reduce the risk of developing bone conditions later in life, such as osteoporosis.

Here are some foods that are rich in calcium:

- Low-fat dairy products

- Cabbage

- Legumes

- Broccoli

- Cauliflower

- Tofu

Now you know the awesome benefits of a healthy balanced diet, I'm sure you are on the edge of your seat waiting to see the healthy and easy to make meals planned out for you. Be sure to try them out and begin eating healthier today.

Enjoy!

BREAKFAST

Berry Cream Compote Over Crepes

Preparation Time: 45 minutes | **Servings:** 8

Per Serving: Calories 339 Fats 24. 5g Carbs 30g Protein 2. 3g

Ingredients:

For the berry cream:
- 2 knob plants butter
- 4 tbsps pure date sugar
- 2 tsps vanilla extract
- 1 cup fresh blueberries
- 1 cup fresh raspberries
- 1 cup whipped coconut cream

For the crepes:
- 4 tbsps flax seed powder + 6 tbsps water
- 2 tsps vanilla extract
- 2 tsps pure date sugar
- ½ tsp salt
- 4 cups almond flour
- 3 cups almond milk
- 3 cups water
- 6 tbsps plant butter for frying

Directions:

1. Melt butter in a pot over low heat and mix in the date sugar and vanilla.
2. Cook until the sugar melts, and then toss in berries. Allow softening for 2 3 minutes.

3. Set aside to cool.
4. In a medium bowl, mix the flax seed powder with water and allow thickening for 5 minutes to make the flax egg. Whisk in the vanilla, date sugar, and salt.
5. Pour in a quarter cup of almond flour and whisk, then a quarter cup of almond milk, and mix until no lumps remain. Repeat the mixing process with the remaining almond flour and almond milk in the same quantities until exhausted.
6. Mix in 1 cup of water until the mixture is runny like that of pancakes, and add the remaining water until the mixture is lighter. Brush a large non-stick skillet with some butter and place over medium heat to melt.
7. Pour 1 tablespoon of the batter into the pan and swirl the skillet quickly and all around to coat the pan with the batter. Cook until the batter is dry and golden brown beneath, about 30 seconds.
8. Use a spatula to carefully flip the crepe and cook the other side until golden brown too. Fold the crepe onto a plate and set it aside. Repeat making more crepes with the remaining batter until exhausted. Plate the crepes, top with the whipped coconut cream and the berry compote.

Serve immediately.

Pimiento Cheese Breakfast Biscuits

Preparation Time: 30 minutes | **Servings:** 8

Per serving: Calories 1009 Fats 71. 8g Carbs 74. 8g Protein 24. 5g

Ingredients:

- 4 cups whole-wheat flour
- 4 tsps baking powder
- 2 tsps salt
- 1 tsp baking soda
- 1 tsp garlic powder
- 1/2 tsp black pepper
- 1/4 cup unsalted plant butter, cold and cut into 1/2-inch cubes
- 3/2 cups of coconut milk
- 2 cups shredded cashew cheese
- 2 (4 oz) jar chopped pimientos, well-drained
- 2 tbsps melted unsalted plant butter

Directions:

1. Preheat the oven to 450 F and line a baking sheet with parchment paper. Set aside. In a medium bowl, mix the flour, baking powder, salt, baking soda, garlic powder, and black pepper. Add the cold butter using a hand mixer until the mixture is the size of small peas.

2. Pour in ¾ of the coconut milk and continue whisking. Continue adding the remaining coconut milk, a tablespoonful at a time, until dough forms.
3. Mix in the cashew cheese and pimientos. (If the dough is too wet to handle, mix in a little bit more flour until it is manageable). Place the dough on a lightly floured surface and flatten the dough into ½-inch thickness.
4. Use a 2 ½-inch round cutter to cut out biscuits' pieces from the dough. Gather, re-roll the dough once and continue cutting out biscuits. Arrange the biscuits on the prepared pan and brush the tops with the melted butter. Bake for 12-14 minutes, or until the biscuits are golden brown. Cool and serve.

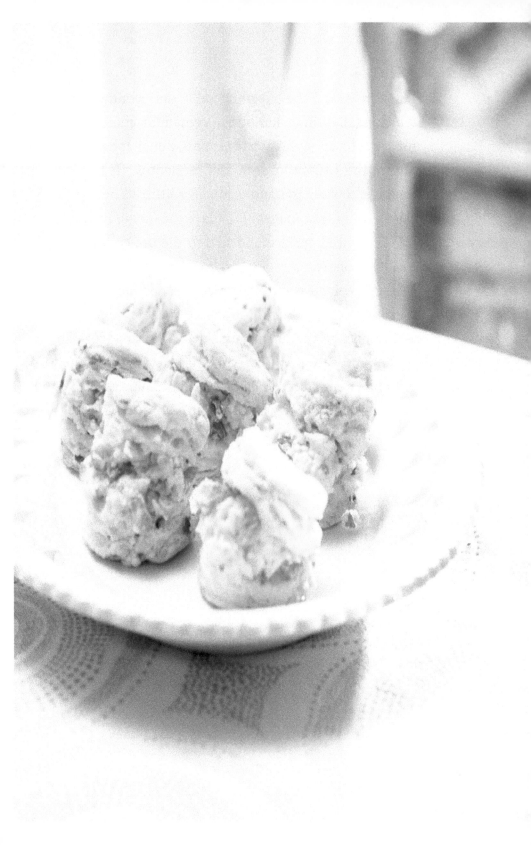

Pumpkin-Pistachio Tea Cake

Preparation Time: 80 minutes | **Servings:** 8

Per Serving: Calories 330 Fats 13. 2g Carbs 50. 1g Protein 7g

Ingredients:

- 4 tbsps flaxseed powder + 6 tbsps water
- 6 tbsps vegetable oil
- 3/2 cups canned unsweetened pumpkin puree
- 1 cup pure corn syrup
- 6 tbsps pure date sugar
- 3 cups whole-wheat flour
- 1 tsp cinnamon powder
- 1 tsp baking powder
- ½ tsp cloves powder
- 1 tsp allspice powder
- 1 tsp nutmeg powder
- A pinch salt
- 4 tbsps chopped pistachios

Directions:

1. Preheat the oven to 350 F and lightly coat an 8 x 4-inch loaf pan with cooking spray. In a medium bowl, mix the flax seed powder with water and allow thickening for 5 minutes to make the flax egg.
2. In a bowl, whisk the vegetable oil, pumpkin puree, corn syrup, date sugar, and flax egg. In another

bowl, mix the flour, cinnamon powder, baking powder, cloves powder, allspice powder, nutmeg powder, and salt. Add this mixture to the wet batter and mix until well combined.

3. Pour the batter into the loaf pan, sprinkle the pistachios on top, and gently press the nuts onto the batter to stick.

4. Bake in the oven for 50 to 55 minutes or until a toothpick inserted into the cake comes out clean. Remove the cake onto a wire rack, allow cooling, slice, and serve.

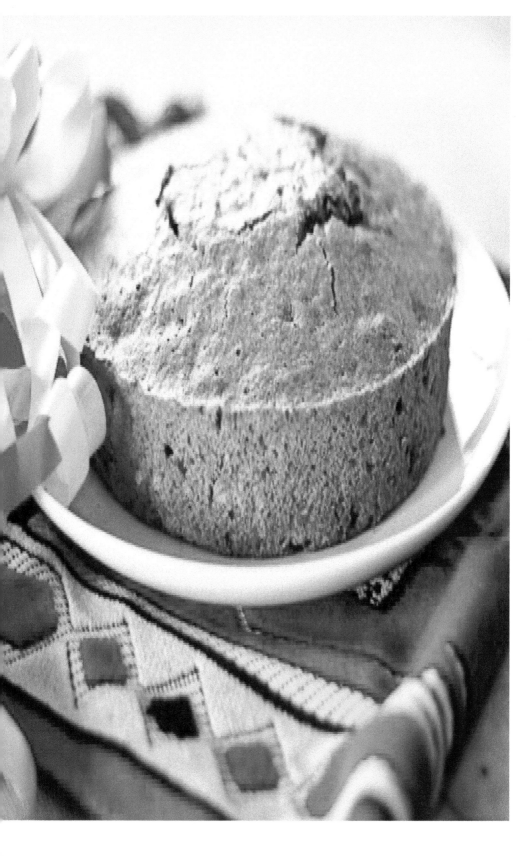

Toasted Rye with Pumpkin Seed Butter

Preparation Time: 30 minutes | **Servings:** 8

Per serving: Carbs: 3 g Protein: 5 g Fats: 10. 3 g Calories: 127 Kcal

Ingredients:
- Pumpkin seeds: 220g Date nectar: 2 tsps
- Avocado oil: 4 tbsps
- Rye bread: 8 slices toasted

Directions:
1. Toast the pumpkin seed on a frying pan on low heat for 5-7 minutes and stir in between
2. Let them turn golden and remove them from the pan
3. Add to the blender when they cool down and make fine powder
4. Add in avocado oil and salt and then again blend to form a paste
5. Add date nectars too and blend
6. On the toasted rye, spread one tablespoon of this butter and serve with your favorite toppings

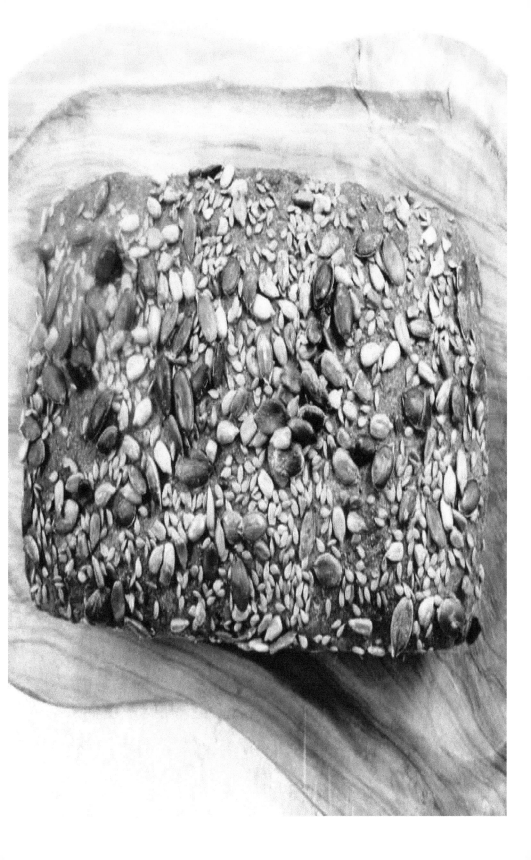

Mushroom & Spinach Chickpea Omelet

Ready in about: 25 minutes | **Servings:** 8

Ingredients

- 2 cups chickpea flour
- 1 tsp onion powder
- 1 tsp garlic powder
- ½ tsp white pepper
- 1/6 cup nutritional yeast
- 1 tsp baking soda
- 2 green bell pepper, chopped
- 6 scallions, chopped
- 2 cups sautéed button mushrooms
- 1 cup chopped fresh spinach
- 2 cups halved cherry tomatoes
- 2 tbsps fresh parsley leaves

Directions

1. In a medium bowl, mix the chickpea flour, onion powder, garlic powder, white pepper, nutritional yeast, and baking soda until well combined.

2. Heat a medium skillet over medium heat and add a quarter of the batter.

3. Swirl the pan to spread the batter across the pan. Scatter a quarter each of the bell pepper, scallions,

mushrooms, and spinach on top and cook until the bottom part of the omelet sets, 1-2 minutes.

4. Carefully flip the omelet and cook the other side until set and golden brown. Transfer the omelet to a plate and make the remaining omelets. Serve the omelet with the tomatoes and garnish with the parsley leaves.

Grandma's Breakfast Gallete

Ready in about: 40 minutes | **Servings:** 5

Per serving: Calories: 208; Fat: 7.7g; Carbs: 27.7g; Protein: 4.8g

Ingredients

- 2 cups all-purpose flour
- 1 cup oat flour
- 2 teaspoons baking powder
- 2 teaspoons baking soda
- 1 teaspoon kosher salt
- 2 teaspoons brown sugar
- 1/2 teaspoon ground allspice
- 2 cups water
- 1 cup rice milk
- 4 tablespoons olive oil

Directions

1. Mix the flour, baking powder, baking soda, salt, sugar and ground allspice using an electric mixer.
2. Gradually pour in the water, milk and oil and continue mixing until everything is well incorporated.
3. Heat a lightly greased griddle over medium-high heat.

4. Ladle 1/4 of the batter into the preheated griddle and cook until your galette is golden and crisp. Repeat with the remaining batter.
5. Serve your galette with homemade jelly, if desired.

Bon appétit!

Breakfast Cranberry and Coconut Crisp

Ready in about: 30 minutes | **Servings:** 10

Per serving: Calories: 209; Fat: 13.5g; Carbs: 26.2g; Protein: 3.5g

Ingredients

- 1 cup rye flakes
- 1 cup rolled oats
- 1 cup spelt flakes
- 1 cup walnut halves
- 2 cups flaked coconut
- 1/6 teaspoon salt
- 1 teaspoon ground cloves
- 1 teaspoon ground cardamom
- 2 teaspoons cinnamon
- 2 teaspoons vanilla extract
- 1/6 cup coconut oil, at room temperature
- 1 cup maple syrup
- 6 cups cranberries

Directions

1. Begin by preheating your oven to 340 degrees. Spritz a baking pan with non-stick oil. Arrange the cranberries in the bottom of your pan.
2. Mix the remaining ingredients until everything is well incorporated. Spread the mixture over the cranberries.

3. Bake in the preheated oven for about 35 minutes or until the top is golden brown.
4. Serve at room temperature.

Bon appétit!

Grandma's Breakfast Waffles

Ready in about: 20 minutes | **Servings:** 8

Per serving: Calories: 316; Fat: 9.9g; Carbs: 50.4g; Protein: 8.3g

Ingredients

- 2 cups all-purpose flour
- 1 cup spelt flour
- 2 teaspoons baking powder
- A pinch of salt
- 1/2 teaspoon ground cinnamon
- 1/2 teaspoon grated nutmeg
- 1 teaspoon vanilla extract
- 2 cups almond milk, unsweetened
- 4 tablespoons blackstrap molasses
- 4 tablespoons coconut oil, melted
- 2 tablespoons fresh lime juice

Directions

1. Preheat a waffle iron according to the manufacturer's instructions.
2. In a mixing bowl, thoroughly combine the flour, baking powder, salt, cinnamon, nutmeg and vanilla extract.
3. In another bowl, mix the liquid ingredients. Then, gradually add in the wet mixture to the dry mixture.
4. Beat until everything is well blended.

5. Ladle 1/4 of the batter into the preheated waffle iron and cook until the waffles are golden and crisp. Repeat with the remaining batter.
6. Serve your waffles with a fruit compote or coconut cream, if desired.

Bon appétit!

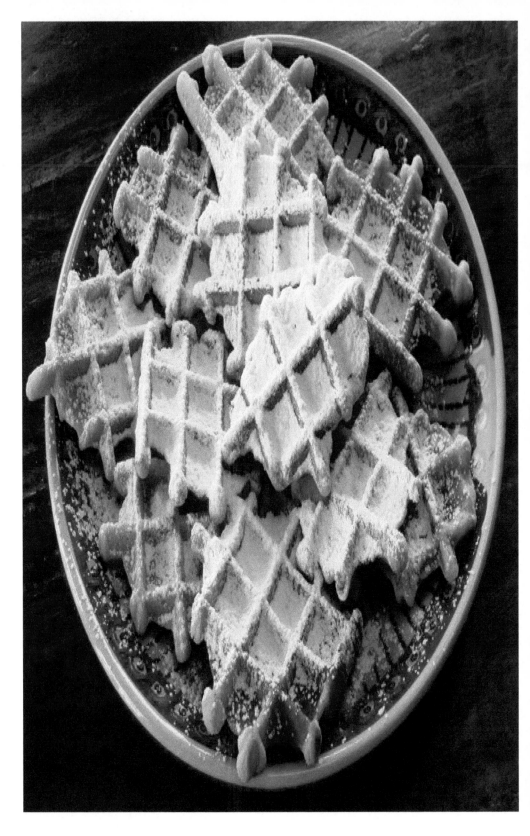

Classic Breakfast Burrito

Ready in about: 15 minutes | **Servings:** 8

Per serving: Calories: 593; Fat: 23.7g; Carbs: 71.7g; Protein: 30.4g

Ingredients

- 2 tablespoons olive oil
- 32 ounces tofu, pressed
- 8 (6-inch) whole-wheat tortillas
- 3 cups canned chickpeas, drained
- 2 medium-sized avocado, pitted and sliced
- 2 tablespoons lemon juice
- 2 teaspoons garlic, pressed
- 4 bell peppers, sliced
- Sea salt and ground black pepper, to taste
- 1 teaspoon red pepper flakes

Directions

1. Heat the olive oil in a frying skillet over medium heat. When it's hot, add the tofu and sauté for about 10 minutes, occasionally stirring to promote even cooking.
2. Divide the fried tofu between warmed tortillas; place the remaining ingredients on your tortillas, roll them up and serve immediately.

Bon appétit!

Homemade Toast Crunch

Ready in about: 15 minutes | **Servings:** 16

Per serving: Calories: 330; Fat: 25.7g; Carbs: 24.7g; Protein: 4.8g

Ingredients

- 2 cups almond flour
- 2 cups coconut flour
- 1 cup all-purpose flour
- 2 cups sugar
- 2 teaspoons kosher salt
- 2 teaspoons cardamom
- 1/2 teaspoon grated nutmeg
- 2 tablespoons cinnamon
- 6 tablespoons flax seeds, ground
- 1 cup coconut oil, melted
- 16 tablespoons coconut milk

Directions

1. Begin by preheating the oven to 340 degrees F. In a mixing bowl, thoroughly combine all the dry ingredients.
2. Gradually pour in the oil and milk; mix to combine well.
3. Shape the dough into a ball and roll it out between 2 sheets of parchment paper. Cut into small

squares and prick them with a fork to prevent air bubbles.

4. Bake in the preheated oven for about 15 minutes. They will continue to crisp as they cool. Bon appétit!

LUNCH

Spicy Cauliflower Pasta

Ready in about: 15 minutes | **Servings:** 4

Per serving: Calories298, Total Fat 10. 4g, Saturated Fat 7. 2g, Cholesterol 50mg, Sodium 426mg, Total Carbohydrate 39. 6g, Dietary Fiber 1. 5g, Total Sugars 1. 8g, Protein 12. 2g

Ingredients:

- 2 tablespoons coconut oil
- 2 teaspoons garlic powder
- ½ teaspoon paprika
- 1 cup cauliflower florets
- 1 cup broccoli florets
- 2 cups bow tie pasta
- Salt & pepper to taste
- 2 cups vegetable broth

Directions:

1. In the Instant Pot, set the Sauté button and add coconut oil when oil is hot; place garlic powder, paprika, cauliflower florets, broccoli florets, salt, and pepper.
2. Sauté the mixture until it's cooked thoroughly.
3. Add the vegetable broth and dry bow tie pasta.
4. Mix very well and place the lid on the Instant Pot, and bring the toggle switch into the "Sealing" position.

5. Press Manual or Pressure Cook and adjust the time for 5 minutes.
6. When the five minutes are up, do a Natural-release for 5 minutes and then move the toggle switch to "Venting" to release the rest of the pressure in the pot.
7. Remove the lid. If the mixture looks watery, press "Sauté", and bring the mixture up to a boil and let it boil for a few minutes. It will thicken as it boils.

Serve and enjoy!

Kale Lasagna Roll-Ups

Ready in about: 25 minutes | **Servings:** 4

Per serving: Calories 343, Total Fat 23. 6g, Saturated Fat 22. 1g, Cholesterol 17. 5mg, Sodium 243mg, Total Carbohydrate 16. 2g, Dietary Fiber 3. 6g, Total Sugars 2. 2g, Protein 16. 4g

Ingredients:

- 1 cup Lasagna noodles
- 1 cup goat cheese
- 1 cup mozzarella, shredded
- 2 large eggs
- ½ cup kale
- 1 cup marinara sauce
- Salt and pepper to taste
- Enough water

Directions:

1. Set Instant Pot to Sauté. Add the kale with goat cheese, mozzarella, egg, pepper, and salt. Stir regularly.
2. Add marinara sauce, water, noodles. Mix well. Stir to make sure noodles are covered with the liquid.
3. Lock the lid and make sure the vent is closed. Set Instant Pot to Manual or Pressure Cook on High Pressure for 15 minutes. When cooking time ends,

release pressure and wait for steam to completely stop before opening the lid.

4. If you would like to sprinkle a bit on top of the Lasagna when you serve it.

Creamy Tofu Marsala Pasta

Ready in about: 25 minutes | **Servings:** 4

Per Serving: Calories 510, Total Fat 20. 6g, Saturated Fat 14. 8g, Cholesterol 7mg, Sodium 432mg, Total Carbohydrate 45. 9g, Dietary Fiber 4. 8g, Total Sugars 7. 8g, Protein 19. 1g

Ingredients:

- ½ cup butter
- 2 tablespoons coconut oil
- 2 small onions, diced
- 4 cups mushrooms, sliced
- 1 cup tofu, diced into chunks
- 1 teaspoon garlic powder
- 3 cups of vegetable broth
- 2 cups of white wine
- 1 cup sun-dried tomatoes
- 2 cups fusilli
- 1/2 cup coconut cream
- 1 cup grated goat cheese

Directions:

1. Add the butter to the Instant Pot. Hit "Sauté".
2. Add the onion and mushrooms and cook for 3-5 minutes until the mushrooms have softened and browned a bit.

3. Then, add the tofu and the coconut oil from the sun-dried tomatoes and cook for another 2-3 minutes until the tofu is slightly white.
4. Toss in the garlic powder and cook for 1 more minute and then add in the white wine and let it simmer for 1 minute more.
5. Add in the vegetable broth and stir together well.
6. Pour in the fusilli so it's laying on top of the broth, gently smoothing and pushing it down with a spatula so it's submerged, but do not stir it with the rest of the broth.
7. Secure the lid and hit "Manual" or "Pressure Cook" High Pressure for 6 minutes. Quick-release when done and give it all a good stir.
8. Stir in the coconut cream and goat cheese. Let it sit for about 5 minutes, stirring occasionally, and it will thicken up into an incredible sauce, coating all the pasta perfectly.
9. Transfer to a serving bowl, plate it up and sprinkle any extra goat cheese if desired.

Enjoy!

Decadent Bread Pudding with Apricots

Ready in about: 1 hour | **Servings:** 8

Per serving: Calories: 418; Fat: 18.8g; Carbs: 56.9g; Protein: 7.3g

Ingredients

- 8 cups day-old ciabatta bread, cubed
- 8 tablespoons coconut oil, melted
- 4 cups coconut milk
- 1 cup coconut sugar
- 8 tablespoons applesauce
- 1/2 teaspoon ground cloves
- 1 teaspoon ground cinnamon
- 2 teaspoons vanilla extract
- 1/6 cup dried apricots, diced

Directions

1. Start by preheating your oven to 360 degrees F. Lightly oil a casserole dish with a non-stick cooking spray.
2. Place the cubed bread in the prepared casserole dish.
3. In a mixing bowl, thoroughly combine the coconut oil, milk, coconut sugar, applesauce, ground cloves, ground cinnamon and vanilla. Pour the custard evenly over the bread cubes; fold in the apricots.

4. Press with a wide spatula and let it soak for about 15 minutes.
5. Bake in the preheated oven for about 45 minutes or until the top is golden and set.

Bon appétit!

Chipotle Cilantro Rice

Ready in about: 25 minutes | **Servings:** 4

Per serving: Calories: 313; Fat: 15g; Carbs: 37.1g; Protein: 5.7g

Ingredients

- 8 tablespoons olive oil
- 2 chipotle pepper, seeded and chopped
- 2 cups jasmine rice
- 3 cups vegetable broth
- 1/2 cup fresh cilantro, chopped
- Sea salt and cayenne pepper, to taste

Directions

1. In a saucepan, heat the olive oil over a moderately high flame. Add in the pepper and rice and cook for about 3 minutes or until aromatic.
2. Pour the vegetable broth into the saucepan and bring to a boil; immediately turn the heat to a gentle simmer.
3. Cook for about 18 minutes or until all the liquid has absorbed. Fluff the rice with a fork, add in the cilantro, salt and cayenne pepper; stir to combine well.

Bon appétit!

Oat Porridge with Almonds

Ready in about: 20 minutes | **Servings:** 2

Per serving: Calories: 533; Fat: 13.7g; Carbs: 85g; Protein: 21.6g

Ingredients

- 2 cups of water
- 4 cups almond milk, divided
- 2 cups rolled oats
- 4 tablespoons coconut sugar
- 1 vanilla essence
- 1/2 teaspoon cardamom
- 1 cup almonds, chopped
- 2 bananas, sliced

Directions

1. In a deep saucepan, bring the water and milk to a rapid boil. Add in the oats, cover the saucepan and turn the heat to medium.
2. Add in the coconut sugar, vanilla and cardamom. Continue to cook for about 12 minutes, stirring periodically.
3. Spoon the mixture into serving bowls; top with almonds and banana.

Bon appétit!

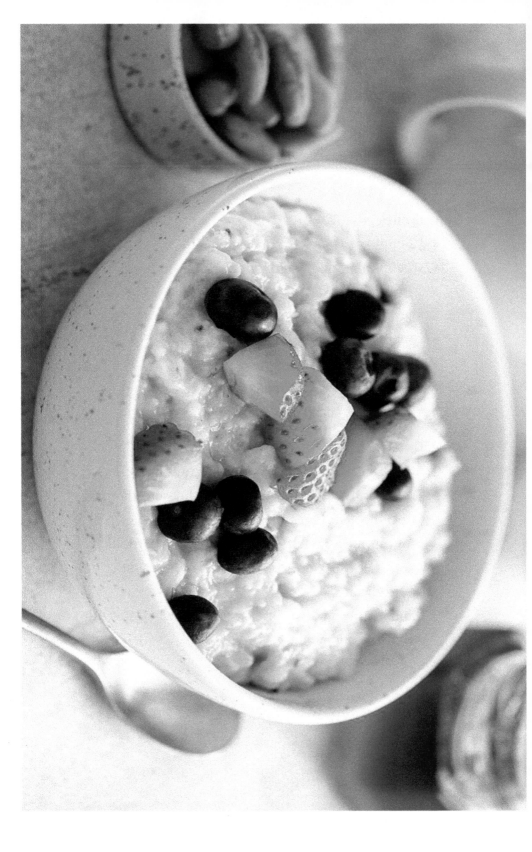

Harissa Bulgur Bowl

Ready in about: 25 minutes | **Servings:** 8

Per serving: Calories: 353; Fat: 15.5g; Carbs: 48.5g; Protein: 8.4g

Ingredients

- 2 cups bulgur wheat
- 3 cups vegetable broth
- 4 cups sweet corn kernels, thawed
- 2 cups canned kidney beans, drained
- 2 red onions, thinly sliced
- 2 garlic cloves, minced
- Sea salt and ground black pepper, to taste
- 1/2 cup harissa paste
- 2 tablespoons lemon juice
- 2 tablespoons white vinegar
- 1/2 cup extra-virgin olive oil
- 1/2 cup fresh parsley leaves, roughly chopped

Directions

1. In a deep saucepan, bring the bulgur wheat and vegetable broth to a simmer; let it cook, covered, for 12 to 13 minutes.
2. Let it stand for 5 to 10 minutes, and fluff your bulgur with a fork.
3. Add the remaining ingredients to the cooked bulgur wheat; serve warm or at room temperature.

Bon appétit!

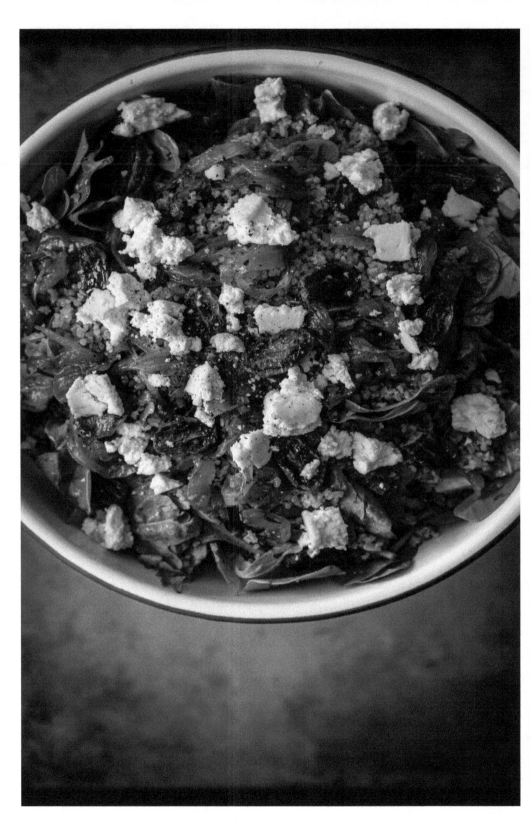

Coconut Quinoa Pudding

Ready in about: 20 minutes | **Servings:** 6

Per serving: Calories: 391; Fat: 10.6g; Carbs: 65.2g; Protein: 11.1g

Ingredients

- 2 cups water
- 2 cups coconut milk
- 2 cups quinoa
- A pinch of kosher salt
- A pinch of ground allspice
- 1 teaspoon cinnamon
- 1 teaspoon vanilla extract
- 8 tablespoons agave syrup
- 1 cup coconut flakes

Directions

1. Place the water, coconut milk, quinoa, salt, ground allspice, cinnamon and vanilla extract in a saucepan.
2. Bring it to a boil over medium-high heat. Turn the heat to a simmer and let it cook for about 20 minutes; fluff with a fork and add in the agave syrup.
3. Divide between three serving bowls and garnish with coconut flakes.

Bon appétit!

Cremini Mushroom Risotto

Ready in about: 20 minutes | **Servings:** 6

Per serving: Calories: 513; Fat: 12.5g; Carbs: 88g; Protein: 11.7g

Ingredients

- 6 tablespoons vegan butter
- 2 teaspoons garlic, minced
- 2 teaspoons thyme
- 2-pound Cremini mushrooms, sliced
- 3 cups white rice
- 5 cups vegetable broth
- 1/2 cup dry sherry wine
- Kosher salt and ground black pepper, to taste
- 6 tablespoons fresh scallions, thinly sliced

Directions

1. In a saucepan, melt the vegan butter over a moderately high flame. Cook the garlic and thyme for about 1 minute or until aromatic.
2. Add in the mushrooms and continue to sauté until they release the liquid or about 3 minutes.
3. Add in the rice, vegetable broth and sherry wine. Bring to a boil; immediately turn the heat to a gentle simmer.

4. Cook for about 15 minutes or until all the liquid has absorbed. Fluff the rice with a fork, season with salt and pepper and garnish with fresh scallions.

Bon appétit!

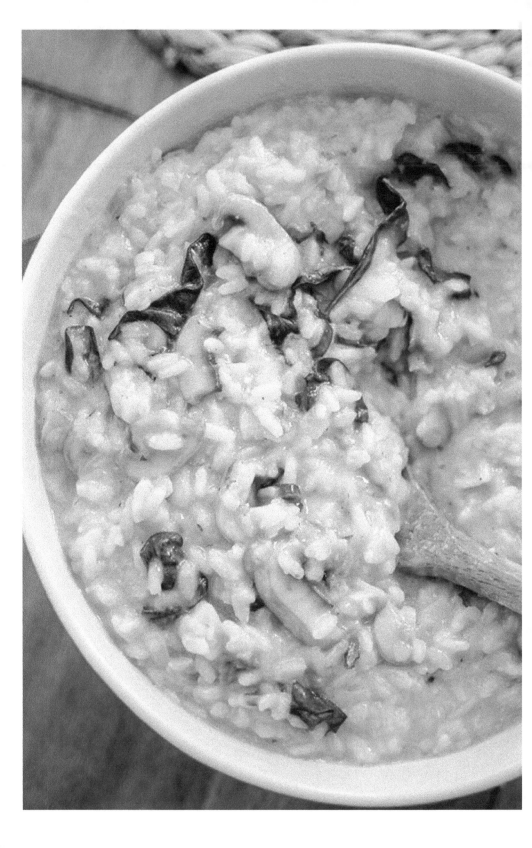

Colorful Risotto with Vegetables

Ready in about: 35 minutes | **Servings:** 10

Per serving: Calories: 363; Fat: 7.5g; Carbs: 66.3g; Protein: 7.7g

Ingredients

- 4 tablespoons sesame oil
- 2 onions, chopped
- 4 bell peppers, chopped
- 2 parsnips, trimmed and chopped
- 2 carrots, trimmed and chopped
- 2 cups broccoli florets
- 4 garlic cloves, finely chopped
- 1 teaspoon ground cumin
- 4 cups brown rice
- Sea salt and black pepper, to taste
- 1 teaspoon ground turmeric
- 4 tablespoons fresh cilantro, finely chopped

Directions

1. Heat the sesame oil in a saucepan over medium-high heat.
2. Once hot, cook the onion, peppers, parsnip, carrot and broccoli for about 3 minutes until aromatic.
3. Add in the garlic and ground cumin; continue to cook for 30 seconds more until aromatic.
4. Place the brown rice in a saucepan and cover it with cold water by 2 inches. Bring to a boil. Turn

the heat to a simmer and continue to cook for about 30 minutes or until tender.

5. Stir the rice into the vegetable mixture; season with salt, black pepper and ground turmeric; garnish with fresh cilantro and serve immediately

Bon appétit!

DINNER

Mushroom, Vegetable, And Rice Curry

Ready in about: 38 minutes | **Servings:** 12

Per serving: Calories 174, Total Fat 10g, Saturated Fat 2g, Total Carbs 23g, Net Carbs 15g, Protein 7g, Sugar: 7g, Fiber: 8g, Sodium: 147mg, Potassium: 968mg, Phosphorus: 450mg

Ingredients:

- 2 tablespoons olive oil
- 4 cloves garlic, minced
- 2 onion, chopped
- 2 fresh chili, chopped
- 2 teaspoons turmeric powder
- 2 teaspoons fenugreek seeds
- 2 teaspoons black mustard seeds
- 2 teaspoons curry powder
- 1 pounds mixed mushrooms sliced
- 1 pounds of mixed vegetables
- 1 cup brown basmati rice
- 2 14-ounce coconut milk
- salt and pepper to taste
- 1 cup of water
- A bunch of fresh coriander, chopped

Directions:

1. Press the Sauté button on the Instant Pot and heat the oil. Sauté the garlic and onion for a minute. Stir in the chili, turmeric powder, fenugreek seeds,

mustard seeds, and curry powder. Stir for another minute or until toasted.

2. Stir in the mushrooms and stir for 3 minutes or until wilted.
3. Stir in the rest of the ingredients except for the coriander.
4. Close the lid and do not seal the vent.
5. Press the Rice button and cook using the preset cooking time.
6. Once cooked, stir in the coriander last.

Smoky Veggie Chili

Read in about: 37 minutes | **Servings:** 10

Per serving: Calories 586, Total Fat 4g, Saturated Fat 0.7g, Total Carbs 126g, Net Carbs 108g, Protein 15g, Sugar: 14g, Fiber: 18g, Sodium: 123mg, Potassium: 3131mg, Phosphorus: 426mg

Ingredients:
- 2 tablespoons olive oil
- 4 onions, chopped
- 2 teaspoons cumin seeds
- 4 teaspoons smoked paprika
- 4 teaspoons cocoa powder
- 2 tablespoons peanut butter
- 2 fresh chili, chopped
- 6 mixed color peppers, seeded and chopped
- 6 large tomatoes, chopped
- 4 sweet potatoes, peeled and cubed
- 16 small jacket potatoes
- 2 bunch fresh coriander, chopped
- salt and pepper to taste
- 2 cups of water

Directions:
1. Press the Sauté button on the Instant Pot and heat the oil.
2. Sauté the onions and cumin until fragrant.

3. Stir in the paprika, cocoa powder, peanut butter, chili, peppers, tomatoes, and potatoes.
4. Season with salt and pepper and pour in water.
5. Close the lid and set the vent to the Sealing position.
6. Press the Meat/Stew button and cook using the preset cooking time.
7. Do natural pressure release.

Sicilian Aubergine Stew

Ready in about: 30 minutes | **Servings:** 10

Per serving: Calories 161, Total Fat 10g, Saturated Fat 1g, Total Carbs 9g, Net Carbs 7g, Protein 10g, Sugar: 3g, Fiber: 2g, Sodium: 131mg, Potassium: 323mg, Phosphorus: 99mg

Ingredients:

- 4 tablespoons olive oil
- 2 small onions, chopped
- 6 cloves garlic, minced
- 2 large aubergine, chopped
- 4 large tomatoes, chopped
- 2 tablespoons caper
- 16 green olives, pitted
- 2 tablespoons red wine vinegar
- 1 cup couscous
- salt and pepper to taste
- 6 cups of water
- 2 tablespoons flaked almonds

Directions:

1. Press the Sauté button and heat the olive oil. Sauté the onion and garlic until fragrant.
2. Stir in the aubergine and tomatoes for three minutes until slightly wilted.

3. Add the capers, olives, red wine vinegar, and couscous. Season with salt and pepper to taste. Pour water.
4. Close the lid and set the vent to the Sealing position.
5. Press the Meat/Stew button and adjust the cooking time to 20 minutes.
6. Do natural pressure release.
7. Once the lid is open, sprinkle with flaked almonds.

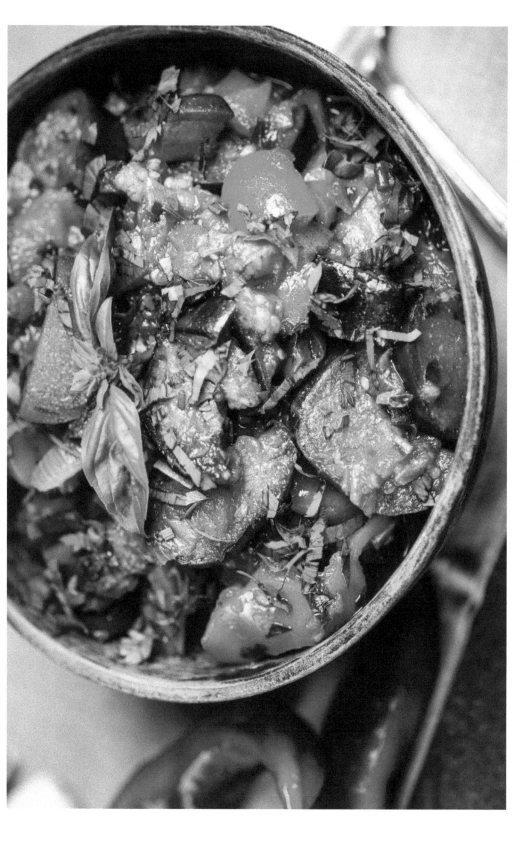

Aubergine Dip

Ready in about: 20 minutes | **Servings:** 4

Per serving: Calories 102, Total Fat 4g, Saturated Fat 0.5g, Total Carbs 18g, Net Carbs: 9 g, Protein 3g, Sugar: 10g, Fiber: 9g, Sodium: 66mg, Potassium: 662mg, Phosphorus: 72mg

Ingredients:

- 2 large aubergines
- 2 cloves garlic, minced
- 2 fresh green chili, minced
- 2 tablespoons extra-virgin olive oil
- Juice from 1 lemon
- 1 teaspoon smoked paprika
- salt and pepper to taste

Directions:

1. Pour water into the Instant Pot and place a trivet or steamer basket inside.
2. Place the aubergine inside.
3. Close the lid and set the vent to the Sealing position.
4. Press the Steam button and cook for 10 minutes.
5. Do natural pressure release.
6. Remove the aubergine from the Instant Pot and allow it to cool.

7. Once cooled, peel the aubergine and place it in a food processor.
8. Add the rest of the ingredients. Pulse until smooth.
9. Serve with crackers.

Walnut Lentil Burgers

Ready in about: 70 minutes |**Serving:** 4

Ingredients

- 2 tbsps olive oil
- 1 cup dry lentils, rinsed
- 2 carrots, grated
- 1 onion, diced
- ½ cup walnuts
- 1 tbsp tomato puree
- ¾ cup almond flour
- 2 tsps curry powder
- 4 whole-grain buns

Directions

1. Place lentils in a pot and cover them with water. Bring to a boil and simmer for 15-20 minutes.

2. Meanwhile, combine the carrots, walnuts, onion, tomato puree, flour, curry powder, salt, and pepper in a bowl. Toss to coat. Once the lentils are ready, drain and transfer them into the veggie bowl. Mash the mixture until sticky. Shape the mixture into balls; flatten to make patties.

3. Heat the oil in a skillet over medium heat. Brown the patties for 8 minutes on both sides. To assemble, put the cakes on the buns and top with your desired toppings.

Couscous & Quinoa Burgers

Ready in about: 20 minutes |**Servings:** 4

Ingredients

- 4 tbsps olive oil
- ½ cup couscous
- ½ cup boiling water
- 4 cups cooked quinoa
- 4 tbsps balsamic vinegar
- 6 tbsps chopped olives
- 1 tsp garlic powder
- Salt to taste
- 8 burger buns
- Lettuce leaves, for serving
- Tomato slices, for serving

Directions

1. Preheat oven to 350 F.

2. In a bowl, place the couscous with boiling water. Let sit covered for 5 minutes. Once the liquid is absorbed, fluff with a fork. Add in quinoa and mash them to form a chunky texture. Stir in vinegar, olive oil, olives, garlic powder, and salt.

3. Shape the mixture into 4 patties. Arrange them on a greased tray and bake for 25-30 minutes. To assemble, place the patties on the buns and top with lettuce and tomato slices. Serve.

Moroccan Lentil and Raisin Salad

Ready in about 20 minutes + chilling time | Servings 8
Per serving: **Calories: 418; Fat: 15g; Carbs: 62.9g; Protein: 12.4g**

Ingredients

- 2 cups red lentils, rinsed
- 2 large carrots, julienned
- 2 Persian cucumbers, thinly sliced
- 2 sweet onions, chopped
- 1 cup golden raisins
- 1/2 cup fresh mint, snipped
- 1/2 cup fresh basil, snipped
- 1/2 cup extra-virgin olive oil
- 1/2 cup lemon juice, freshly squeezed
- 2 teaspoons grated lemon peel
- 1 teaspoon fresh ginger root, peeled and minced
- 1 teaspoon granulated garlic
- 2 teaspoons ground allspice
- Sea salt and ground black pepper, to taste

Directions

1. In a large-sized saucepan, bring 3 cups of water and 1 cup of the lentils to a boil.
2. Immediately turn the heat to a simmer and continue to cook your lentils for a further 15 to 17 minutes or until they've softened but are not mushy yet. Drain and let it cool completely.

3. Transfer the lentils to a salad bowl; add in the carrot, cucumber and sweet onion. Then, add the raisins, mint and basil to your salad.
4. In a small mixing dish, whisk the olive oil, lemon juice, lemon peel, ginger, granulated garlic, allspice, salt and black pepper.
5. Dress your salad and serve well-chilled.

Bon appétit!

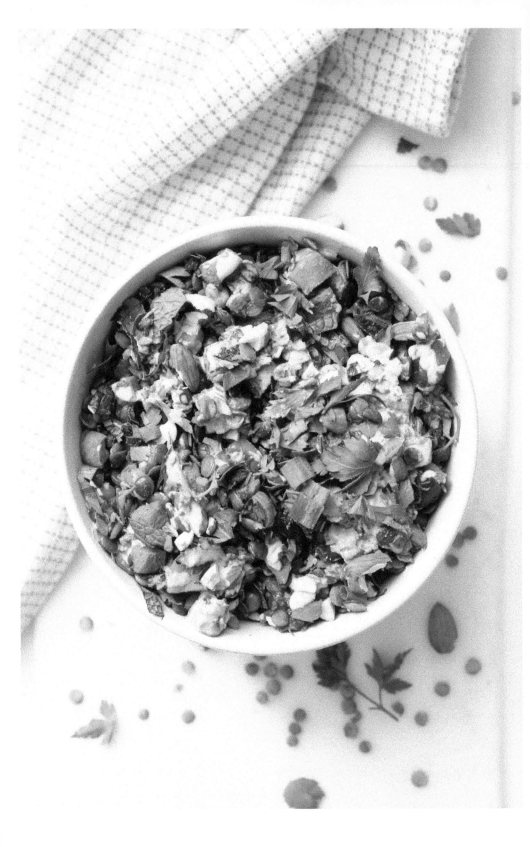

Asparagus and Chickpea Salad

Ready in about: 10 minutes + chilling time | **Servings:** 10
Per serving: Calories: 198; Fat: 12.9g; Carbs: 17.5g;
Protein: 5.5g

Ingredients

- 5/2 pounds asparagus, trimmed and cut into bite-sized pieces
- 10 ounces canned chickpeas, drained and rinsed
- 1 chipotle pepper, seeded and chopped
- 2 Italian peppers, seeded and chopped
- 1/2 cup fresh basil leaves, chopped
- 1/2 cup fresh parsley leaves, chopped
- 4 tablespoons fresh mint leaves
- 4 tablespoons fresh chives, chopped
- 2 teaspoons garlic, minced
- 1/2 cup extra-virgin olive oil
- 2 tablespoons balsamic vinegar
- 2 tablespoons fresh lime juice
- 4 tablespoons soy sauce
- 1/2 teaspoon ground allspice
- 1/2 teaspoon ground cumin
- Sea salt and freshly cracked peppercorns, to taste

Directions

1. Bring a large pot of salted water with the asparagus to a boil; let it cook for 2 minutes; drain and rinse.

2. Transfer the asparagus to a salad bowl.
3. Toss the asparagus with chickpeas, peppers, herbs, garlic, olive oil, vinegar, lime juice, soy sauce and spices.
4. Toss to combine and serve immediately.

Bon appétit!

Old-Fashioned Green Bean Salad

Ready in about: 10 minutes + chilling time | **Servings:** 8
Per serving: Calories: 240; Fat: 14.1g; Carbs: 29g;
Protein: 4.4g

Ingredients

1. 3 pounds green beans, trimmed
2. 1 cup scallions, chopped
3. 2 teaspoons garlic, minced
4. 2 Persian cucumbers, sliced
5. 4 cups grape tomatoes, halved
6. ½ cup olive oil
7. 2 teaspoons deli mustard
8. 4 tablespoons tamari sauce
9. 4 tablespoons lemon juice
10. 2 tablespoons apple cider vinegar
11. ½ teaspoon cumin powder
12. 1 teaspoon dried thyme
13. Sea salt and ground black pepper, to taste

Directions

1. Boil the green beans in a large saucepan of salted water until they are just tender or about 2 minutes.
2. Drain and let the beans cool completely; then, transfer them to a salad bowl. Toss the beans with the remaining ingredients.

Bon appétit!

Winter Bean Soup

Ready in about: 25 minutes | **Servings:** 8

Per serving: Calories: 234; Fat: 5.5g; Carbs: 32.3g; Protein: 14.4g

Ingredients

1. 2 tablespoons olive oil
2. 4 tablespoons shallots, chopped
3. 2 carrots, chopped
4. 2 parsnips, chopped
5. 2 celeries stalk, chopped
6. 2 teaspoons fresh garlic, minced
7. 8 cups vegetable broth
8. 4 bay leaves
9. 2 rosemary sprigs, chopped
10. 32 ounces canned navy beans
11. Flaky sea salt and ground black pepper, to taste

Directions

1. In a heavy-bottomed pot, heat the olive over medium-high heat. Now, sauté the shallots, carrot, parsnip and celery for approximately 3 minutes or until the vegetables are just tender.
2. Add in the garlic and continue to sauté for 1 minute or until aromatic.
3. Then, add in the vegetable broth, bay leaves and rosemary and bring to a boil. Immediately reduce the heat to a simmer and let it cook for 10 minutes.

4. Fold in the navy beans and continue to simmer for about 5 minutes longer until everything is thoroughly heated. Season with salt and black pepper to taste.
5. Ladle into individual bowls, discard the bay leaves and serve hot.

Bon appétit!

DESSERT

Roasted Asparagus with Sesame Seeds

Ready in about: 25 minutes | **Servings:** 8

Per serving: Calories: 215; Fat: 19.1g; Carbs: 8.8g; Protein: 5.6g

Ingredients

- 3 pounds asparagus, trimmed
- 8 tablespoons extra-virgin olive oil
- Sea salt and ground black pepper, to taste
- 1 teaspoon dried oregano
- 1 teaspoon dried basil
- 2 teaspoons red pepper flakes, crushed
- 8 tablespoons sesame seeds
- 4 tablespoons fresh chives, roughly chopped

Directions

1. Start by preheating the oven to 400 degrees F. Then, line a baking sheet with parchment paper.
2. Toss the asparagus with olive oil, salt, black pepper, oregano, basil and red pepper flakes. Now, arrange your asparagus in a single layer on the prepared baking sheet.
3. Roast your asparagus for approximately 20 minutes.
4. Sprinkle sesame seeds over your asparagus and continue to bake an additional 5 minutes or until

the asparagus spears are crisp-tender and the sesame seeds are lightly toasted.

5. Garnish with fresh chives and serve warm.

Bon appétit!

Aromatic Sautéed Swiss Chard

Ready in about: 15 minutes | **Servings:** 8

Per serving: Calories: 124; Fat: 6.7g; Carbs: 11.1g; Protein: 5g

Ingredients

- 4 tablespoons vegan butter
- 2 onions, chopped
- 4 cloves garlic, sliced
- Sea salt and ground black pepper, to season
- 3 pounds Swiss chard, torn into pieces, tough stalks removed
- 2 cups vegetable broth
- 2 bay leafs
- 2 thyme sprigs
- 4 rosemary sprigs
- 1 teaspoon mustard seeds
- 2 teaspoons celery seeds

Directions

1. In a saucepan, melt the vegan butter over medium-high heat.
2. Then, sauté the onion for about 3 minutes or until tender and translucent; sauté the garlic for about 1 minute until aromatic.
3. Add in the remaining ingredients and turn the heat to a simmer; let it simmer, covered, for about 10 minutes or until everything is cooked through.

Bon appétit!

Mediterranean-Style Green Beans

Ready in about: 20 minutes | **Servings:** 8
Per serving: Calories: 159; Fat: 8.8g; Carbs: 18.8g;
Protein: 4.8g

Ingredients

- 4 tablespoons olive oil
- 2 red bell peppers, seeded and diced
- 3 pounds green beans
- 8 garlic cloves, minced
- 1 teaspoon mustard seeds
- 1 teaspoon fennel seeds
- 2 teaspoons dried dill weed
- 4 tomatoes, pureed
- 2 cups cream of celery soup
- 2 teaspoons Italian herb mix
- 2 teaspoons cayenne pepper
- Salt and freshly ground black pepper

Directions

1. Heat the olive oil in a saucepan over medium flame. Once hot, fry the peppers and green beans for about 5 minutes, stirring periodically to promote even cooking.
2. Add in the garlic, mustard seeds, fennel seeds and dill and continue sautéing an additional 1 minute or until fragrant.

3. Add in the pureed tomatoes, cream of celery soup, Italian herb mix, cayenne pepper, salt and black pepper. Continue to simmer, covered, for about 9 minutes or until the green beans are tender.
4. Taste, adjust the seasonings and serve warm.

Bon appétit!

Vanilla Cookies with Poppy Seeds

Ready in about: 15 minutes | **Servings:** 6

Ingredients

- 3/2 cups plant butter, softened
- 1 cup pure date sugar
- 2 tsps pure vanilla extract
- 4 tbsps pure maple syrup
- 4 cups whole-grain flour
- 3/2 cups poppy seeds, lightly toasted

Directions

1. Beat the butter and sugar in a bowl until creamy and fluffy. Add in vanilla, and maple syrup, blend. Stir in flour and poppy seeds. Wrap the dough in a cylinder and cover it with plastic foil. Let chill in the fridge.

2. Preheat oven to 330 F. Cut the dough into thin circles and arrange on a baking sheet. Bake for 12 minutes until light brown. Let completely cool before serving.

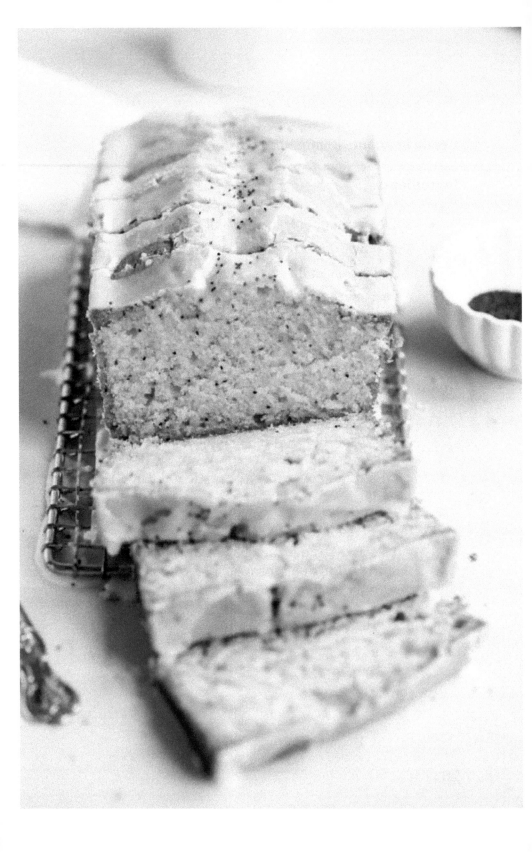

Kiwi & Peanut Bars

Ready in about: 5 minutes |**Servings:** 9

Ingredients

- 4 kiwis, mashed
- 2 tbsps maple syrup
- 1 tsp vanilla extract
- 4 cups old-fashioned rolled oats
- 1 tsp salt
- ½ cup chopped peanuts

Directions

1. Preheat oven to 360 F.

2. In a bowl, add kiwi, maple syrup, and vanilla and stir. Mix in oats, salt, and peanuts. Pour into a greased baking dish and bake for 25-30 minutes until crisp. Let completely cool and slice into bars to serve.

Tropical Cheesecake

Ready in about: 20 minutes + cooling time |**Servings:** 8

Ingredients

- 2/3 cup toasted rolled oats
- ¼ cup plant butter, melted
- 3 tbsps pure date sugar
- 6 oz cashew cream cheese
- ¼ cup coconut milk
- 1 lemon, zested and juiced
- ¼ cup just-boiled water
- 3 tsps agar agar powder
- 1 ripe mango, chopped

Directions

1. Process the oats, butter, and date sugar in a blender until smooth.

2. Pour the mixture into a greased 9-inch springform pan and press the mixture onto the bottom of the pan. Refrigerate for 30 minutes until firm while you make the filling.

3. In a large bowl, using an electric mixer, whisk the cashew cream cheese until smooth. Beat in the coconut milk, lemon zest, and lemon juice. Mix the boiled water and agar agar powder until dissolved and whisk this mixture into the creamy mix. Fold in the mango.

4. Remove the cake pan from the fridge and pour in the mango mixture. Shake the pan to ensure smooth layering on top. Refrigerate further for at least 3 hours. Remove the cheesecake from the fridge, release the cake pan, slice, and serve.

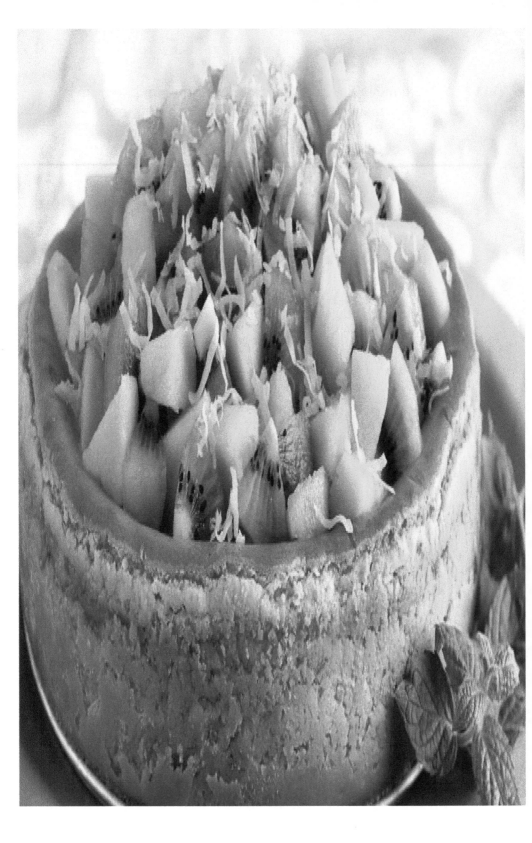

Keto Brownies

Ready in about: 30minutes | **Servings:** 4

Per serving: Calories: 321, Total Fat: 40.3g, Saturated Fat: 18 g, Total Carbs: 19 g, Dietary Fiber: 5g, Sugar: 4 g, Protein: 2 g, Sodium: 265 mg

Ingredients:

- 4 tbsps flax seed powder + 6 tbsps water
- ½ cup unsweetened cocoa powder
- 1 cup almond flour
- 1 tsp baking powder
- 1 cup erythritol
- 20 tablespoons butter 1 cup + 4 tbsps
- 4 oz dairy-free dark chocolate
- 1 teaspoon vanilla extract optional

Directions:

1. Preheat the oven to 375 F and line a baking sheet with parchment paper. Set aside.
2. Mix the flaxseed powder with water in a bowl and allow thickening for 5 minutes.
3. In a separate bowl, mix the cocoa powder, almond flour, baking powder, and erythritol until no lumps from the erythritol remain.
4. In another bowl, add the butter and dark chocolate and melt both in the microwave for 30 seconds to 1 minute.

5. Whisk the flax egg and vanilla into the chocolate mixture, then pour the mixture into the dry ingredients. Combine evenly.
6. Pour the batter onto the paper-lined baking sheet and bake in the oven for 20 minutes or until a toothpick inserted into the cake comes out clean.
7. Remove from the oven to cool completely and refrigerate for 30 minutes to 2 hours.
8. When ready, slice into squares, and serve.

Ambrosia Salad with Pecans

Ready in about:15 minutes + 1-hour chilling | **Servings:** 8

Per serving: Calories 648 Fats 36g Carbs 85. 7g Protein 6. 6g

Ingredients:
- 2 cups pure coconut cream
- 1 tsp vanilla extract
- 4 medium bananas, peeled and cut into chunks
- 3 cups unsweetened coconut flakes
- 8 tbsps toasted pecans, chopped
- 2 cups pineapple tidbits, drained
- 2 (11 oz) can mandarin oranges, drained
- 3/2 cups maraschino cherries stems removed

Directions:
1. In a medium bowl, mix the coconut cream and vanilla extract until well combined.
2. In a larger bowl, combine the bananas, coconut flakes, pecans, pineapple, oranges, and cherries until evenly distributed.
3. Pour on the coconut cream mixture and fold well into the salad.
4. Chill in the refrigerator for 1 hour and serve afterwards.

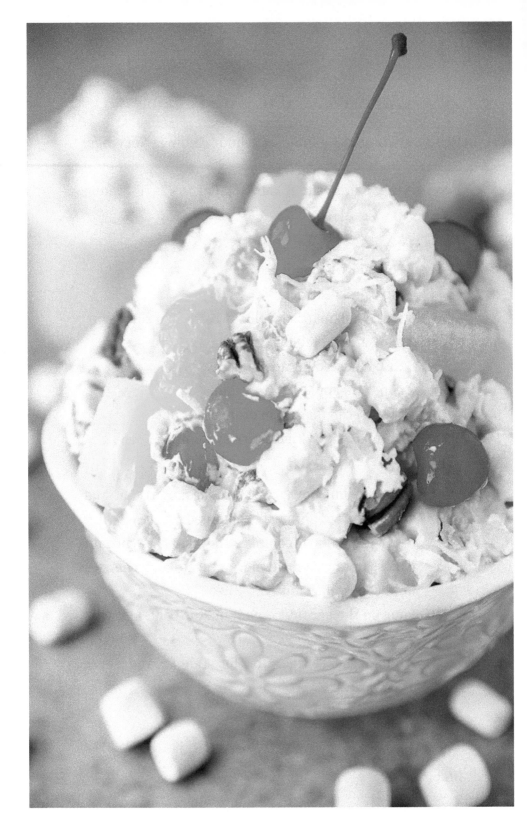

Chocolate and Avocado Pudding

Ready in about: 3 hours and 10 minutes | **Servings:** 2

Per serving: Calories: 87 Cal Fat: 7 g Carbs: 9 g Protein: 1.5 g Fiber: 3.2 g

Ingredients:

- 2 small avocados, pitted, peeled
- 2 small bananas, mashed
- 1/6 cup cocoa powder, unsweetened
- 2 tablespoons cacao nibs, unsweetened
- 1/2 cup maple syrup
- 1/6 cup coconut cream

Directions:

1. Add avocado in a food processor along with cream and then pulse for 2 minutes until smooth.
2. Add remaining ingredients, blend until mixed, and then tip the pudding in a container.
3. Cover the container with a plastic wrap; it should touch the pudding and refrigerate for 3 hours.
4. Serve straight away.

Chocolate Avocado Ice Cream

Preparation Time: 1 hour and 10 minutes | **Servings:** 4

Per serving: Calories: 80.7 Cal Fat: 7.1 g Carbs: 6 g Protein: 0.6 g Fiber: 2 g

Ingredients:

- 8 ounces avocado, peeled, pitted
- 1 cup cocoa powder, unsweetened
- 2 tablespoons vanilla extract, unsweetened
- 1 cup and 2 tablespoons maple syrup
- 26 ounces coconut milk, unsweetened
- 1 cup water

Directions:

1. Add avocado in a food processor along with milk and then pulse for 2 minutes until smooth.
2. Add remaining ingredients, blend until mixed, and then tip the pudding in a freezer-proof container.
3. Place the container in a freezer and chill for freeze for 4 hours until firm, whisking every 20 minutes after 1 hour.

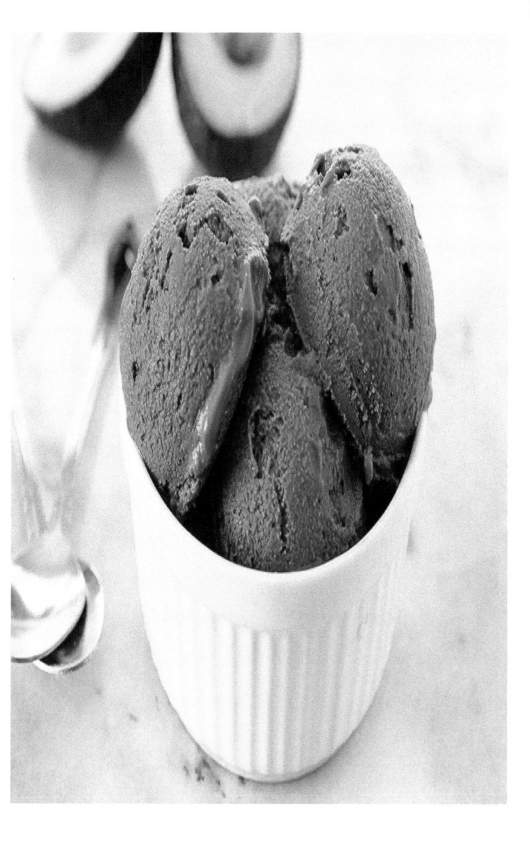

SNACKS

Spiced Roasted Cauliflower

Ready in about: 25 minutes | **Servings:** 12
Per serving: Calories: 115; Fat: 9.3g; Carbs: 6.9g; Protein: 5.6g

Ingredients

- 3 pounds cauliflower florets
- 1/2 cup olive oil
- 8 tablespoons apple cider vinegar
- 4 cloves garlic, pressed
- 2 teaspoons dried basil
- 2 teaspoons dried oregano
- Sea salt and ground black pepper, to taste

Directions

1. Begin by preheating your oven to 420 degrees F.
2. Toss the cauliflower florets with the remaining ingredients.
3. Arrange the cauliflower florets on a parchment-lined baking sheet. Bake the cauliflower florets in the preheated oven for about 25 minutes or until they are slightly charred.

Bon appétit!

Tofu Stuffed Peppers

Ready in about: 25 minutes |**Serving:** 8

Ingredients

- 2 cups red and yellow bell peppers
- 2 oz tofu, chopped into small bits
- 2 cups cashew cream cheese
- 2 tbsps chili paste, mild
- 4 tbsps melted plant butter
- 2 cups grated plant-based Parmesan

Directions

1. Preheat oven to 400 F. Use a knife to cut the bell peppers into two (lengthwise) and remove the core.

2. In a bowl, mix tofu, cashew cream cheese, chili paste, and melted butter until smooth. Spoon the cheese mixture into the bell peppers and use the back of the spoon to level the filling in the peppers. Grease a baking sheet with cooking spray and arrange the stuffed peppers on the sheet.

3. Sprinkle the plant-based Parmesan cheese on top and bake the peppers for 15-20 minutes until the peppers are golden brown and the cheese melted. Remove onto a serving platter and serve warm.

Crispy Squash Nacho Chips

Ready in about: 26 minutes |**Serving:** 8

Ingredients

- 2 large yellow squashes
- 3 cups coconut oil
- 2 tbsps taco seasoning

Directions

1. With a mandolin slicer, cut the squash into thin, round slices and place it in a colander.

2. Sprinkle the squash with a lot of salt and allow sitting for 5 minutes. After, press the water out of the squash and pat dry with a paper towel. Pour the coconut oil into a deep skillet and heat the oil over medium heat.

3. Carefully add the squash slices in the oil, about 20 pieces at a time, and fry until crispy and golden brown. Use a slotted spoon to remove the squash onto a paper towel-lined plate. Sprinkle the slices with taco seasoning and serve.

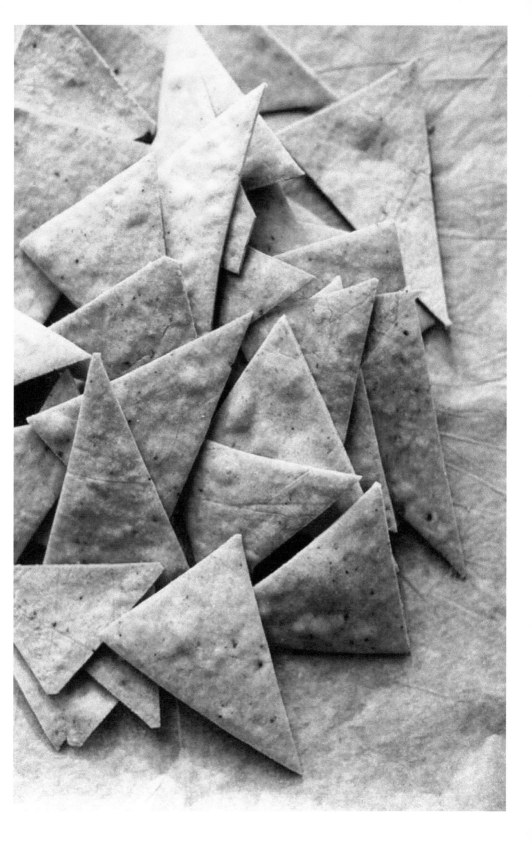

Flavorful Sweet Potatoes with Apples

Ready in about: 5 hours | **Servings:** 12

Per serving: Calories:120 Cal, Carbohydrates:24g, Protein:1g, Fats:3g, Fiber:2g.

Ingredients:

- 6 medium-sized apples, peeled and cored
- 12 medium-sized sweet potatoes, peeled and cored
- 1/2 cup of pecans
- 1/2 teaspoon of ground cinnamon
- 1/2 teaspoon of ground nutmeg
- 4 tablespoons of vegan butter, melted
- 1/2 cup of maple syrup

Directions:

1. Cut the sweet potatoes and the apples into 1/2 inch slices.

2. Grease a 6-quarts slow cooker with a non-stick cooking spray and arrange the sweet potato slices in the bottom of the cooker.

3. Top it with the apple slices; sprinkle it with the cinnamon and nutmeg before garnishing it with butter.

4. Cover it with the lid, plug in the slow cooker and let it cook on the low heat setting for 4 hours or until the sweet potatoes get soft.
5. When done, sprinkle it with pecans and continue cooking for another 30 minutes.

Serve right away.

Buttery Baby Potatoes

Ready in about: 40 minutes | **Servings:** 8

Per serving: Calories 192 kcal Fats 8. 8g Carbs 25. 7g Protein 4. 1g

Ingredients:
- 8 tbsps unsalted plant butter, melted
- 8 garlic cloves, minced
- 6 tbsps chopped chives
- Salt and black pepper to taste
- 4 tbsps grated plant-based Parmesan cheese
- 3 lbs. baby potatoes, rinsed and drained

Directions:
1. Preheat the oven to 400 F.
2. In a large bowl, mix the butter, garlic, chives, salt, black pepper, and plant Parmesan cheese. Toss the potatoes in the butter mixture until well coated.
3. Spread the mixture into a baking sheet, cover with foil, and roast in the oven for 30 minutes or until tender.
4. Remove the potatoes from the oven and toss in the remaining butter mixture. Serve.

Sweetened Carrots with Parsley Drizzle

Ready in about: 14 minutes | **Servings:** 8

Per serving: Calories 120 kcal Fats 6g Carbs 16. 8g Protein 1. 1g

Ingredients:
- 2 lbs. baby carrots
- 4 tbsps plant butter
- 4 tbsps pure maple syrup
- 2 tbsps freshly squeezed lemon juice
- 1 tsp black pepper
- ½ cup chopped fresh parsley

Directions:
1. Boil some water in a medium pot. Add some salt and cook the carrots until tender, 5 to 6 minutes. Drain the carrots.
2. Melt the butter in a large skillet and mix in the maple syrup and lemon juice.
3. Toss in the carrots, season with black pepper, and toss in the parsley.
4. Serve the carrots.

Chipotle and Lime Tortilla Chips

Ready in about: 15 minutes | **Servings:** 8

Per serving: Calories: 150 Cal Fat: 7 g Carbs: 18 g Protein: 2 g Fiber: 2 g

Ingredients:

- 12 ounces whole-wheat tortillas
- 4 tablespoons chipotle seasoning 1 tablespoon olive oil
- 4 limes, juiced

Directions:

1. Whisk together oil and lime juice, brush it well on tortillas, then sprinkle with chipotle seasoning and bake for 15 minutes at 350 degrees F until crispy, turning halfway.
2. When done, let the tortilla cool for 10 minutes, then break it into chips and serve.

Easy Lebanese Toum

Ready in about: 10 minutes | **Servings:** 12
Per serving: Calories: 252; Fat: 27g; Carbs: 3.1g; Protein: 0.4g

Ingredients

- 4 heads garlic
- 2 teaspoons coarse sea salt
- 3 cups olive oil
- 2 lemons, freshly squeezed
- 4 cups carrots, cut into matchsticks

Directions

1. Puree the garlic cloves and salt in your food processor of a high-speed blender until creamy and smooth, scraping down the sides of the bowl.
2. Gradually and slowly, add in the olive oil and lemon juice, alternating between these two ingredients to create a fluffy sauce.
3. Blend until the sauce has thickened. Serve with carrot sticks and enjoy!

Avocado with Tangy Ginger Dressing

Ready in about: 10 minutes | **Servings:** 8

Per serving: Calories: 295; Fat: 28.2g; Carbs: 11.3g; Protein: 2.3g

Ingredients

- 4 avocados, pitted and halved
- 2 clove garlic, pressed
- 2 teaspoons fresh ginger, peeled and minced
- 4 tablespoons balsamic vinegar
- 8 tablespoons extra-virgin olive oil
- Kosher salt and ground black pepper, to taste

Directions

1. Place the avocado halves on a serving platter.
2. Mix the garlic, ginger, vinegar, olive oil, salt and black pepper in a small bowl. Divide the sauce between the avocado halves.

Bon appétit!

Chickpea Snack Mix

Ready in about: 30 minutes | **Servings:** 16
Per serving: Calories: 109; Fat: 7.9g; Carbs: 7.4g; Protein: 3.4g

Ingredients

- 2 cups roasted chickpeas, drained
- 4 tablespoons coconut oil, melted
- 1/2 cup raw pumpkin seeds
- 1/2 cup raw pecan halves
- 1/6 cup dried cherries

Directions

1. Pat the chickpeas dry using paper towels. Drizzle coconut oil over the chickpeas.
2. Roast the chickpeas in the preheated oven at 380 degrees F for about 20 minutes, tossing them once or twice.
3. Toss your chickpeas with the pumpkin seeds and pecan halves. Continue baking until the nuts are fragrant about 8 minutes; let cool completely.
4. Add in the dried cherries and stir to combine.

Bon appétit!

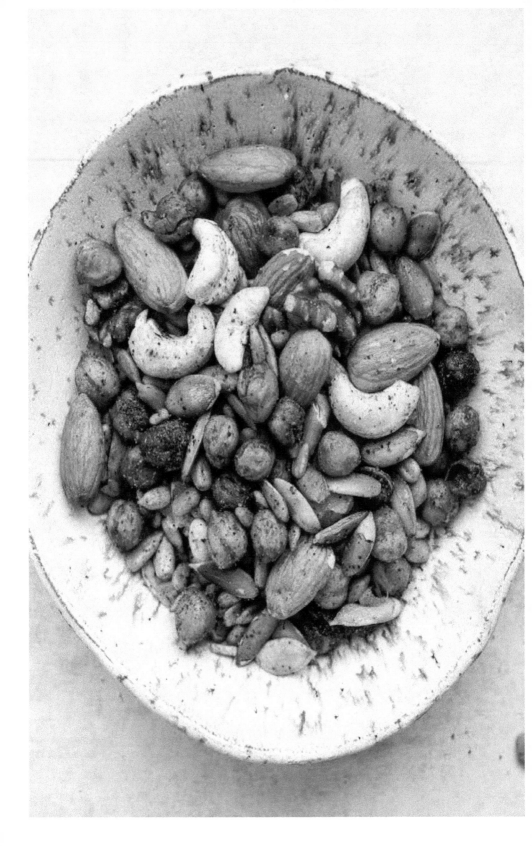

CONCLUSION

There are a plethora of compelling reasons to make a positive difference and transition to a plant-based diet. A plant-based diet will increase your quality of life by providing you with more energy and stamina, assisting you in losing excess body weight, and perhaps even extending your time in this magnificent world. Too much energy and fossil fuels are lost in the process of obtaining meat and other animal products, shipping them over miles and miles of road, and refining them. You will also be bringing a genuine and important difference to the future of our planet Earth by making the transition.

By switching to rich plant-based meals, we can save the earth and also take care of ourselves.

Thank you for taking the time to read this.

Lightning Source UK Ltd.
Milton Keynes UK
UKHW021014030521
383041UK00001B/123